PLANT-BASED RECIPES FOR DIABETICS TO MANAGE BLOOD SUGAR

A Plant-Based Recipe Guide for Managing Diabetes

Isabella Adams

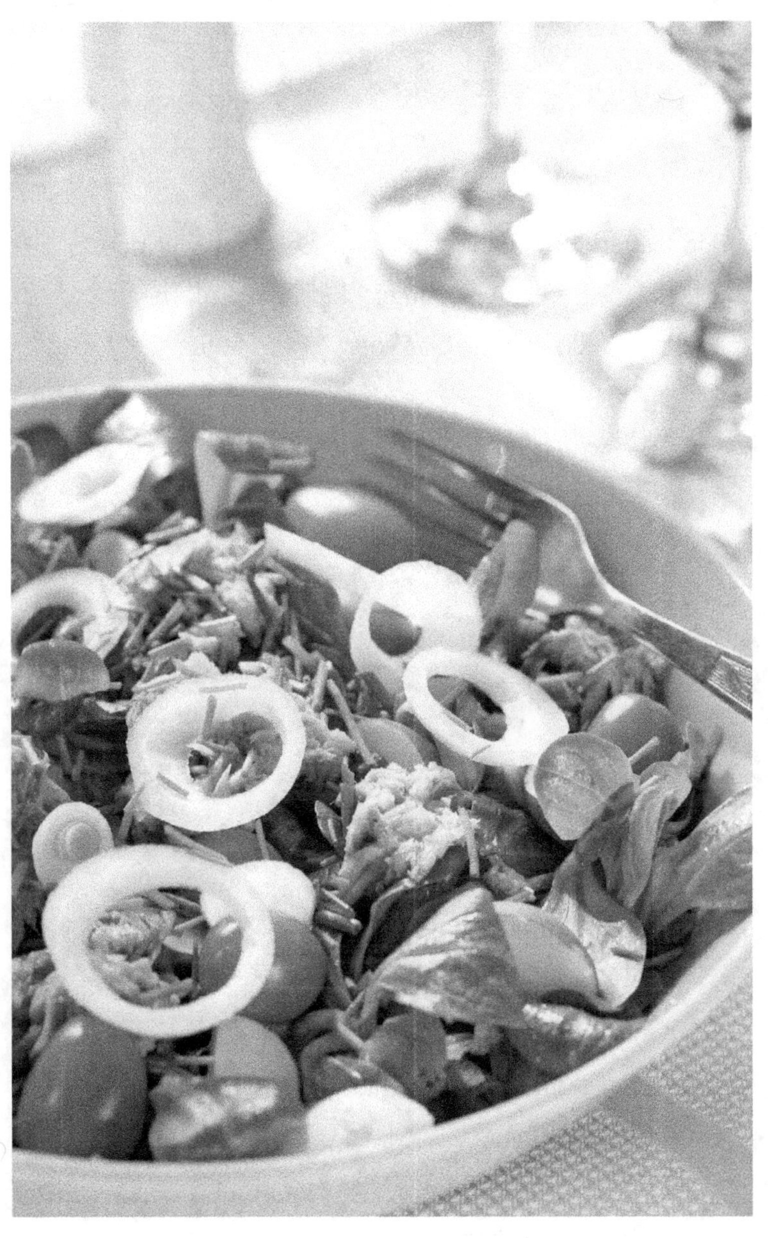

TABLE OF CONTENTS

Chapter 3: Lunch Recipes 45

Chapter 4: Dinner Recipes 71

Chapter 5: Snacks and Appetizers 97

INTRODUCTION

Diabetes can feel like a whirlwind of information and adjustments. But take a deep breath, because you have the power to manage your health through the incredible world of food! Let's break down the role of diet in diabetes control, explore the benefits of plant-based eating, and equip you with tips to rock plant-powered meals.

Understanding Diabetes and the Diet Connection:

Diabetes disrupts how your body uses blood sugar (glucose) for energy. Normally, insulin, a hormone, helps usher glucose into cells. In diabetes, either your body doesn't produce enough insulin, or your cells resist its effects. This leads to high blood sugar levels, which can damage organs over time.

Diet plays a starring role in managing blood sugar. Certain foods cause blood sugar spikes, while others offer a slow, steady release. By making smart choices, you can significantly impact your blood sugar levels and overall diabetes management.

The Plant-Based Advantage:

Plant-based eating, which emphasizes fruits, vegetables, whole grains, legumes, nuts, and seeds, offers a treasure trove of benefits for people with diabetes:

- **Fiber Powerhouse:** Plant foods are packed with fiber, which slows down sugar absorption into your bloodstream, preventing those unwanted spikes.

- **Weight Management Ally:** Plant-based diets tend to be lower in calories and fat, promoting healthy weight loss or maintenance, a crucial factor in diabetes control.

- **Heart-Healthy Benefits:** Many plant-based foods are rich in antioxidants and unsaturated fats, which can help lower bad cholesterol and reduce the risk of heart disease, a common complication of diabetes.

Plant-Based Diabetic Cooking: Your Culinary Adventure Awaits!

Ready to embrace the delicious world of plant-based diabetic cooking? Here are some tips to set you on the path to success:

- **Befriend Whole Grains:** Swap refined grains for brown rice, quinoa, whole-wheat bread, and oats. These provide sustained energy and keep you feeling fuller for longer.
- **The Legume Love Affair**: Beans, lentils, and chickpeas are protein and fiber superstars. Explore them in stews, soups, salads, and even dips!
- **Vegetable Extravaganza:** Roast, steam, stir-fry – unleash your inner veggie artist! Aim for a rainbow of colors on your plate for a variety of nutrients.
- **Fruity Delights:** Choose whole fruits over juices for their fiber content. Experiment with berries, apples, pears, and citrus fruits for a sweet and satisfying treat.

- **Spice Up Your Life**! Herbs and spices add depth of flavor without added sugar or sodium. Explore cuisines from around the world for inspiration.
- **Plan and Prep**: Planning meals and prepping ingredients in advance can be a game-changer. It helps avoid unhealthy choices when hunger strikes.

Remember: Don't be afraid to experiment! There's a world of exciting plant-based recipes waiting to be discovered. Embrace the journey, and celebrate every delicious step towards a healthier you.

Chapter 1: 30 Day Meal Plan

Week 1:

Day 1:

- Breakfast: Oatmeal with Berries and Almonds
- Lunch: Chickpea Salad Wraps
- Dinner: Eggplant Parmesan with Whole Wheat Pasta
- Snack: Hummus and Veggie Sticks
- Dessert: Vegan Chocolate Avocado Mousse

Day 2:

- Breakfast: Avocado Toast with Whole Grain Bread
- Lunch: Lentil Soup with Vegetables
- Dinner: Vegan Chili with Beans and Sweet Potatoes
- Snack: Sliced Apple with Almond Butter
- Dessert: Berry and Banana Nice Cream

Day 3:

- Breakfast: Tofu Scramble with Vegetables
- Lunch: Quinoa Stuffed Bell Peppers
- Dinner: Stuffed Portobello Mushrooms

- Snack: Trail Mix with Nuts and Seeds
- Dessert: Pumpkin Spice Energy Bites

Day 4:

- Breakfast: Chia Seed Pudding with Fresh Fruit
- Lunch: Greek Salad with Tofu Feta
- Dinner: Ratatouille with Quinoa
- Snack: Cucumber and Tomato Bruschetta
- Dessert: Coconut Almond Macaroons

Day 5:

- Breakfast: Quinoa Breakfast Bowl
- Lunch: Spinach and Mushroom Quesadillas
- Dinner: Cauliflower Curry with Brown Rice
- Snack: Veggie Sushi Rolls
- Dessert: Chia Seed Berry Popsicles

Day 6:

- Breakfast: Vegan Breakfast Burrito
- Lunch: Cauliflower Rice Stir-Fry
- Dinner: Spaghetti Squash Primavera
- Snack: Kale Chips

- Dessert: Apple Cinnamon Oat Bars

Day 7:

- Breakfast: Green Smoothie Bowl
- Lunch: Vegan Caesar Salad with Tempeh Bacon
- Dinner: Vegan Shepherd's Pie
- Snack: Stuffed Mini Bell Peppers
- Dessert: Vegan Peanut Butter Cups

Week 2:

Day 8:

- Breakfast: Sweet Potato Hash
- Lunch: Black Bean and Corn Tacos
- Dinner: Lentil Sloppy Joes
- Snack: Spicy Edamame
- Dessert: Lemon Poppy Seed Muffins

Day 9:

- Breakfast: Buckwheat Pancakes with Berry Compote
- Lunch: Sweet Potato and Kale Buddha Bowl
- Dinner: Mushroom and Spinach Vegan Lasagna
- Snack: Vegan Cheese and Crackers

- Dessert: Banana Chocolate Chip Cookies

Day 10:

- Breakfast: Lentil Breakfast Patties
- Lunch: Vegan BLT Sandwiches
- Dinner: Teriyaki Tofu Stir-Fry
- Snack: Avocado Cucumber Rolls
- Dessert: Raspberry Coconut Truffles

Day 11:

- Breakfast: Zucchini Fritters
- Lunch: Thai Peanut Noodle Salad
- Dinner: Butternut Squash Risotto
- Snack: Mediterranean Stuffed Grape Leaves
- Dessert: Almond Butter Banana Bites

Day 12:

- Breakfast: Breakfast Quinoa Porridge
- Lunch: Mediterranean Veggie Wrap
- Dinner: Black Bean Enchiladas
- Snack: Sweet Potato Fries with Spicy Dipping Sauce
- Dessert: Carrot Cake Energy Balls

Day 13:

- Breakfast: Spinach and Mushroom Vegan Quiche
- Lunch: Broccoli and White Bean Soup
- Dinner: Moroccan Chickpea Tagine
- Snack: Baked Tofu Bites
- Dessert: Blueberry Almond Crisp

Day 14:

- Breakfast: Banana Walnut Muffins
- Lunch: Edamame and Avocado Sushi Rolls
- Dinner: Coconut Curry Lentil Soup
- Snack: Hummus and Veggie Sticks
- Dessert: Chocolate Covered Strawberries

Week 3:

Day 15:

- Breakfast: Coconut Yogurt Parfait with Granola
- Lunch: Mexican Quinoa Salad
- Dinner: Vegan Pad Thai
- Snack: Guacamole with Baked Tortilla Chips
- Dessert: Mango Coconut Sorbet

Day 16:

- Breakfast: Oatmeal with Berries and Almonds
- Lunch: Chickpea Salad Wraps
- Dinner: Eggplant Parmesan with Whole Wheat Pasta
- Snack: Hummus and Veggie Sticks
- Dessert: Vegan Chocolate Avocado Mousse

Day 17:

- Breakfast: Avocado Toast with Whole Grain Bread
- Lunch: Lentil Soup with Vegetables
- Dinner: Vegan Chili with Beans and Sweet Potatoes
- Snack: Sliced Apple with Almond Butter
- Dessert: Berry and Banana Nice Cream

Day 18:

- Breakfast: Tofu Scramble with Vegetables
- Lunch: Quinoa Stuffed Bell Peppers
- Dinner: Stuffed Portobello Mushrooms
- Snack: Trail Mix with Nuts and Seeds
- Dessert: Pumpkin Spice Energy Bites

Day 19:

- Breakfast: Chia Seed Pudding with Fresh Fruit
- Lunch: Greek Salad with Tofu Feta
- Dinner: Ratatouille with Quinoa
- Snack: Cucumber and Tomato Bruschetta
- Dessert: Coconut Almond Macaroons

Day 20:

- Breakfast: Quinoa Breakfast Bowl
- Lunch: Spinach and Mushroom Quesadillas
- Dinner: Cauliflower Curry with Brown Rice
- Snack: Veggie Sushi Rolls
- Dessert: Chia Seed Berry Popsicles

Day 21:

- Breakfast: Vegan Breakfast Burrito
- Lunch: Cauliflower Rice Stir-Fry
- Dinner: Spaghetti Squash Primavera
- Snack: Kale Chips
- Dessert: Apple Cinnamon Oat Bars

Week 4:

Day 22:

- Breakfast: Sweet Potato Hash
- Lunch: Black Bean and Corn Tacos
- Dinner: Lentil Sloppy Joes
- Snack: Spicy Edamame
- Dessert: Lemon Poppy Seed Muffins

Day 23:

- Breakfast: Buckwheat Pancakes with Berry Compote
- Lunch: Sweet Potato and Kale Buddha Bowl
- Dinner: Mushroom and Spinach Vegan Lasagna
- Snack: Vegan Cheese and Crackers
- Dessert: Banana Chocolate Chip Cookies

Day 24:

- Breakfast: Lentil Breakfast Patties
- Lunch: Vegan BLT Sandwiches
- Dinner: Teriyaki Tofu Stir-Fry
- Snack: Avocado Cucumber Rolls
- Dessert: Raspberry Coconut Truffles

Day 25:

- Breakfast: Zucchini Fritters
- Lunch: Thai Peanut Noodle Salad
- Dinner: Butternut Squash Risotto
- Snack: Mediterranean Stuffed Grape Leaves
- Dessert: Almond Butter Banana Bites

Day 26:

- Breakfast: Breakfast Quinoa Porridge
- Lunch: Mediterranean Veggie Wrap
- Dinner: Black Bean Enchiladas
- Snack: Sweet Potato Fries with Spicy Dipping Sauce
- Dessert: Carrot Cake Energy Balls

Day 27:

- Breakfast: Spinach and Mushroom Vegan Quiche
- Lunch: Broccoli and White Bean Soup
- Dinner: Moroccan Chickpea Tagine
- Snack: Baked Tofu Bites
- Dessert: Blueberry Almond Crisp

Day 28:

- Breakfast: Banana Walnut Muffins
- Lunch: Edamame and Avocado Sushi Rolls
- Dinner: Coconut Curry Lentil Soup
- Snack: Hummus and Veggie Sticks
- Dessert: Chocolate Covered Strawberries

Day 29:

- Breakfast: Coconut Yogurt Parfait with Granola
- Lunch: Mexican Quinoa Salad
- Dinner: Vegan Pad Thai
- Snack: Guacamole with Baked Tortilla Chips
- Dessert: Mango Coconut Sorbet

Day 30:

- Breakfast: Oatmeal with Berries and Almonds
- Lunch: Chickpea Salad Wraps
- Dinner: Eggplant Parmesan with Whole Wheat Pasta
- Snack: Hummus and Veggie Sticks
- Dessert: Vegan Chocolate Avocado Mousse

Chapter 2: Breakfast Recipes

In this chapter, we present delicious and satisfying breakfast recipes that are plant-based and perfect for diabetics. These recipes are not only packed with flavor but also with essential nutrients to help you start your day on the right foot.

Oatmeal with Berries and Almonds

Ingredients:

- 1/2 cup rolled oats
- 1 cup almond milk
- 1/4 cup mixed berries (strawberries, blueberries, raspberries)
- 1 tablespoon sliced almonds
- 1 teaspoon honey or maple syrup (optional)

Instructions:

1. In a saucepan, bring almond milk to a simmer over medium heat.
2. Stir in rolled oats and cook, stirring occasionally, for about 5 minutes or until oats are tender and creamy.

3. Transfer oatmeal to a bowl and top with mixed berries and sliced almonds.

4. Drizzle with honey or maple syrup if desired.

5. Serve hot and enjoy!

Nutrition Information:

- Calories: 300

- Protein: 9g

- Carbohydrates: 45g

- Fat: 10g

- Fiber: 8g

- Sugar: 10g

- Portion Size: 1 serving

Avocado Toast with Whole Grain Bread

Ingredients:

- 2 slices whole grain bread, toasted

- 1 ripe avocado, mashed

- Salt and pepper to taste

- Red pepper flakes (optional)

- Lemon juice (optional)

Instructions:

1. Spread mashed avocado evenly onto toasted whole grain bread slices.
2. Season with salt, pepper, red pepper flakes, and a squeeze of lemon juice if desired.
3. Serve immediately as a nutritious and satisfying breakfast option.

Nutrition Information:

- Calories: 250
- Protein: 7g
- Carbohydrates: 20g
- Fat: 15g
- Fiber: 8g
- Sugar: 2g
- Portion Size: 1 serving

Tofu Scramble with Vegetables

Ingredients:

- 1/2 block firm tofu, crumbled

- 1/4 cup diced bell peppers (any color)
- 1/4 cup diced onions
- 1/4 cup chopped spinach
- 1/4 teaspoon turmeric powder
- Salt and pepper to taste

Instructions:

1. Heat a non-stick skillet over medium heat and add diced onions and bell peppers. Sauté until softened.
2. Add crumbled tofu to the skillet and sprinkle with turmeric powder, salt, and pepper.
3. Cook for 5-7 minutes, stirring occasionally, until tofu is heated through and slightly golden.
4. Add chopped spinach to the skillet and cook for an additional 2-3 minutes until wilted.
5. Serve hot as a delicious and protein-packed breakfast option.

Nutrition Information:

- Calories: 180
- Protein: 15g
- Carbohydrates: 10g

- Fat: 10g

- Fiber: 5g

- Sugar: 3g

- Portion Size: 1 serving

Chia Seed Pudding with Fresh Fruit

Ingredients:

- 1/4 cup chia seeds

- 1 cup almond milk

- 1 tablespoon maple syrup or honey

- 1/2 teaspoon vanilla extract

- Fresh fruit for topping (such as sliced strawberries, blueberries, or kiwi)

Instructions:

1. In a bowl, mix chia seeds, almond milk, maple syrup (or honey), and vanilla extract.

2. Stir well to combine and let it sit for 5 minutes.

3. Stir the mixture again to break up any clumps of chia seeds.

4. Cover the bowl and refrigerate overnight or for at least 4 hours until the pudding thickens.

5. Serve chilled with fresh fruit toppings.

Nutrition Information:

- Calories: 220
- Protein: 6g
- Carbohydrates: 25g
- Fat: 10g
- Fiber: 12g
- Sugar: 10g
- Portion Size: 1 serving

Quinoa Breakfast Bowl

Ingredients:

- 1/2 cup cooked quinoa
- 1/4 cup almond milk
- 1 tablespoon almond butter
- 1/2 banana, sliced
- 1 tablespoon chopped nuts (such as almonds or walnuts)
- Cinnamon for sprinkling
- Optional: drizzle of honey or maple syrup

Instructions:

1. In a bowl, combine cooked quinoa and almond milk.

2. Stir in almond butter until well incorporated.

3. Top with sliced banana, chopped nuts, and a sprinkle
    of cinnamon.

4. Drizzle with honey or maple syrup if desired.

5. Enjoy this protein-rich and satisfying breakfast
    bowl!

Nutrition Information:

- Calories: 320

- Protein: 10g

- Carbohydrates: 35g

- Fat: 15g

- Fiber: 6g

- Sugar: 8g

- Portion Size: 1 serving

Vegan Breakfast Burrito

Ingredients:

- 1 whole grain tortilla

- 1/2 cup black beans, drained and rinsed

- 1/4 cup diced tomatoes

- 1/4 cup diced bell peppers

- 1/4 cup diced onions

- 1/4 cup chopped spinach

- 2 tablespoons salsa

- Optional: sliced avocado and hot sauce

Instructions:

1. Heat the tortilla in a skillet until warm and pliable.

2. Fill the tortilla with black beans, diced tomatoes, bell peppers, onions, and spinach.

3. Top with salsa and any additional toppings such as sliced avocado and hot sauce.

4. Roll up the tortilla tightly, folding in the sides as you go.

5. Serve immediately as a flavorful and filling breakfast option.

Nutrition Information:

- Calories: 280

- Protein: 10g

- Carbohydrates: 45g

- Fat: 5g

- Fiber: 12g

- Sugar: 5g

- Portion Size: 1 serving

Green Smoothie Bowl

Ingredients:

- 1 ripe banana, frozen

- 1 cup spinach leaves

- 1/2 cup kale leaves, stems removed

- 1/2 cup almond milk

- 1 tablespoon almond butter

- Toppings: sliced strawberries, granola, chia seeds

Instructions:

1. In a blender, combine frozen banana, spinach, kale, almond milk, and almond butter.

2. Blend until smooth and creamy, adding more almond milk if needed to reach desired consistency.

3. Pour the smoothie into a bowl and top with sliced strawberries, granola, and chia seeds.

4. Enjoy this nutrient-packed and refreshing breakfast bowl!

Nutrition Information:

* Calories: 280
* Protein: 8g
* Carbohydrates: 35g
* Fat: 12g
* Fiber: 10g
* Sugar: 12g
* Portion Size: 1 serving

Sweet Potato Hash

Ingredients:

* 1 medium sweet potato, peeled and diced
* 1/4 cup diced bell peppers
* 1/4 cup diced onions
* 1/4 cup black beans, drained and rinsed
* 1/2 teaspoon paprika
* Salt and pepper to taste
* 1 tablespoon olive oil

Instructions:

1. Heat olive oil in a skillet over medium heat.
2. Add diced sweet potato and cook until tender, about 8-10 minutes.
3. Stir in diced bell peppers, onions, black beans, paprika, salt, and pepper.
4. Cook for an additional 5 minutes, until vegetables are softened and lightly browned.
5. Serve hot as a flavorful and filling breakfast option.

Nutrition Information:

- Calories: 220
- Protein: 5g
- Carbohydrates: 30g
- Fat: 8g
- Fiber: 7g
- Sugar: 8g
- Portion Size: 1 serving

Buckwheat Pancakes with Berry Compote

Ingredients:

- 1/2 cup buckwheat flour
- 1/2 teaspoon baking powder
- 1/4 teaspoon cinnamon
- Pinch of salt
- 1/2 cup almond milk
- 1 tablespoon maple syrup
- 1/2 cup mixed berries (strawberries, blueberries, raspberries)
- 1 tablespoon water
- 1 teaspoon lemon juice

Instructions:

1. In a bowl, whisk together buckwheat flour, baking powder, cinnamon, and salt.
2. Stir in almond milk and maple syrup until smooth batter forms.
3. Heat a non-stick skillet over medium heat and lightly grease with cooking spray.

4. Pour batter onto the skillet to form pancakes and cook until bubbles form on the surface, then flip and cook until golden brown.

5. In a small saucepan, combine mixed berries, water, and lemon juice. Cook over medium heat until berries are softened and mixture thickens.

6. Serve pancakes topped with berry compote for a delicious and nutritious breakfast.

Nutrition Information:

- Calories: 280
- Protein: 7g
- Carbohydrates: 45g
- Fat: 8g
- Fiber: 6g
- Sugar: 10g
- Portion Size: 1 serving

Lentil Breakfast Patties

Ingredients:

- 1 cup cooked lentils
- 1/4 cup rolled oats

- 1/4 cup diced onions
- 1/4 cup diced bell peppers
- 1 teaspoon garlic powder
- 1/2 teaspoon cumin
- Salt and pepper to taste
- 1 tablespoon olive oil

Instructions:

1. In a mixing bowl, mash cooked lentils until they form a thick paste.
2. Stir in rolled oats, diced onions, bell peppers, garlic powder, cumin, salt, and pepper until well combined.
3. Form mixture into patties using your hands.
4. Heat olive oil in a skillet over medium heat and cook patties until golden brown on both sides, about 3-4 minutes per side.
5. Serve hot as a protein-rich and satisfying breakfast option.

Nutrition Information:

- Calories: 220
- Protein: 12g

- Carbohydrates: 30g
- Fat: 6g
- Fiber: 10g
- Sugar: 3g
- Portion Size: 1 serving

Zucchini Fritters

Ingredients:

- 2 cups grated zucchini
- 1/4 cup chickpea flour
- 1/4 cup nutritional yeast
- 1/4 cup chopped fresh parsley
- 1 teaspoon garlic powder
- Salt and pepper to taste
- Olive oil for frying

Instructions:

1. Place grated zucchini in a clean kitchen towel and squeeze out excess moisture.
2. In a mixing bowl, combine grated zucchini, chickpea flour, nutritional yeast, chopped parsley, garlic powder, salt, and pepper.

3. Heat olive oil in a skillet over medium heat.

4. Form zucchini mixture into small patties and place them in the skillet.

5. Cook for 3-4 minutes on each side until golden brown and crispy.

6. Serve hot as a delicious and nutritious breakfast option.

Nutrition Information:

- Calories: 180
- Protein: 8g
- Carbohydrates: 20g
- Fat: 8g
- Fiber: 6g
- Sugar: 5g
- Portion Size: 1 serving

Breakfast Quinoa Porridge

Ingredients:

- 1/2 cup cooked quinoa
- 1/2 cup almond milk
- 1/2 banana, mashed

- 1 tablespoon almond butter
- 1/4 teaspoon cinnamon
- 1 tablespoon chopped nuts (such as almonds or walnuts)
- Optional: drizzle of honey or maple syrup

Instructions:

1. In a saucepan, combine cooked quinoa and almond milk.
2. Stir in mashed banana, almond butter, and cinnamon.
3. Cook over medium heat until heated through and creamy, about 5 minutes.
4. Pour porridge into a bowl and top with chopped nuts.
5. Drizzle with honey or maple syrup if desired.
6. Enjoy this protein-packed and satisfying breakfast option!

Nutrition Information:

- Calories: 300
- Protein: 9g
- Carbohydrates: 35g
- Fat: 12g

- Fiber: 7g

- Sugar: 8g

- Portion Size: 1 serving

Spinach and Mushroom Vegan Quiche

Ingredients:

- 1 pre-made whole wheat pie crust

- 1 cup silken tofu

- 1 tablespoon nutritional yeast

- 1 tablespoon olive oil

- 1/2 cup diced onions

- 1 cup sliced mushrooms

- 2 cups fresh spinach

- 1/4 teaspoon garlic powder

- Salt and pepper to taste

Instructions:

1. Preheat the oven to 375°F (190°C).

2. In a skillet, heat olive oil over medium heat. Add diced onions and cook until translucent.

3. Add sliced mushrooms and cook until they release their moisture and start to brown.

4. Stir in fresh spinach and cook until wilted. Season with garlic powder, salt, and pepper.

5. In a blender, combine silken tofu and nutritional yeast until smooth.

6. Pour tofu mixture into the pre-made pie crust.

7. Top with the cooked spinach and mushroom mixture.

8. Bake in the preheated oven for 25-30 minutes, or until the quiche is set and lightly golden on top.

9. Allow to cool slightly before slicing and serving.

Nutrition Information:
- Calories: 220
- Protein: 10g
- Carbohydrates: 20g
- Fat: 12g
- Fiber: 5g
- Sugar: 3g
- Portion Size: 1 slice

Banana Walnut Muffins

Ingredients:

- 1 1/2 cups whole wheat flour
- 1 teaspoon baking powder
- 1/2 teaspoon baking soda
- 1/4 teaspoon salt
- 2 ripe bananas, mashed
- 1/4 cup maple syrup
- 1/4 cup almond milk
- 1/4 cup chopped walnuts
- 1 tablespoon ground flaxseeds mixed with 3 tablespoons water (as egg replacer)
- 1 teaspoon vanilla extract

Instructions:

1. Preheat the oven to 350°F (175°C) and line a muffin tin with paper liners.
2. In a large bowl, whisk together whole wheat flour, baking powder, baking soda, and salt.
3. In another bowl, mix mashed bananas, maple syrup, almond milk, flaxseed mixture, and vanilla extract.

4. Pour the wet ingredients into the dry ingredients and mix until just combined.

5. Fold in chopped walnuts.

6. Divide the batter evenly among the muffin cups.

7. Bake for 18-20 minutes, or until a toothpick inserted into the center comes out clean.

8. Allow muffins to cool in the tin for 5 minutes before transferring to a wire rack to cool completely.

Nutrition Information:

- Calories: 180
- Protein: 5g
- Carbohydrates: 25g
- Fat: 8g
- Fiber: 4g
- Sugar: 10g
- Portion Size: 1 muffin

Coconut Yogurt Parfait with Granola

Ingredients:

- 1/2 cup coconut yogurt
- 1/4 cup granola (choose a low-sugar option)

- 1/4 cup mixed berries (such as strawberries, blueberries, raspberries)

Instructions:

1. In a serving glass or bowl, layer coconut yogurt, granola, and mixed berries.
2. Repeat the layers until the glass or bowl is full.
3. Serve immediately as a nutritious and satisfying breakfast parfait.

Nutrition Information:

- Calories: 250
- Protein: 5g
- Carbohydrates: 30g
- Fat: 10g
- Fiber: 6g
- Sugar: 12g
- Portion Size: 1 serving

Chapter 3: Lunch Recipes

In this chapter, we've curated mouthwatering lunch recipes that are not only satisfying but also packed with plant-based goodness. From vibrant salads to hearty wraps and comforting soups, each recipe offers a delightful blend of flavors and textures to tantalize your taste buds.

Chickpea Salad Wraps

Ingredients:

- 1 can (15 ounces) chickpeas, drained and rinsed
- 1/2 cup diced cucumber
- 1/2 cup diced tomato
- 1/4 cup diced red onion
- 2 tablespoons chopped fresh parsley
- 2 tablespoons lemon juice
- 1 tablespoon olive oil
- Salt and pepper to taste
- 4 whole grain tortillas
- Handful of spinach leaves

Instructions:

1. In a large bowl, mash the chickpeas with a fork until slightly chunky.
2. Add cucumber, tomato, red onion, parsley, lemon juice, olive oil, salt, and pepper. Mix well.
3. Place a handful of spinach leaves in the center of each tortilla.
4. Spoon the chickpea salad mixture onto the spinach leaves.
5. Roll up the tortillas tightly, tucking in the sides as you go.
6. Slice each wrap in half and serve.

Nutrition Information:

- Calories: 250
- Protein: 9g
- Carbohydrates: 42g
- Fat: 6g
- Fiber: 8g
- Sugar: 4g
- Portion Size: 1 wrap

Lentil Soup with Vegetables

Ingredients:

- 1 cup dried lentils, rinsed
- 4 cups vegetable broth
- 1 onion, chopped
- 2 carrots, diced
- 2 celery stalks, diced
- 2 cloves garlic, minced
- 1 teaspoon dried thyme
- 1 teaspoon dried rosemary
- Salt and pepper to taste
- Fresh parsley for garnish

Instructions:

1. In a large pot, combine lentils, vegetable broth, onion, carrots, celery, garlic, thyme, and rosemary.
2. Bring to a boil, then reduce heat and simmer for 25-30 minutes until lentils are tender.
3. Season with salt and pepper to taste.
4. Ladle the soup into bowls, garnish with fresh parsley, and serve.

Nutrition Information:

- Calories: 220
- Protein: 14g
- Carbohydrates: 38g
- Fat: 1g
- Fiber: 15g
- Sugar: 6g
- Portion Size: 1 cup

Quinoa Stuffed Bell Peppers

Ingredients:

- 4 bell peppers, any color
- 1 cup quinoa, cooked
- 1 can (15 ounces) black beans, drained and rinsed
- 1 cup corn kernels
- 1 cup diced tomatoes
- 1/2 cup diced red onion
- 1 teaspoon cumin
- 1 teaspoon chili powder
- Salt and pepper to taste
- 1/2 cup shredded vegan cheese (optional)
- Fresh cilantro for garnish

Instructions:

1. Preheat the oven to 375°F (190°C).

2. Cut the tops off the bell peppers and remove the seeds and membranes.

3. In a large bowl, combine cooked quinoa, black beans, corn, tomatoes, red onion, cumin, chili powder, salt, and pepper.

4. Spoon the quinoa mixture into the bell peppers.

5. Place the stuffed peppers in a baking dish and sprinkle with shredded vegan cheese if desired.

6. Cover the baking dish with foil and bake for 25-30 minutes until the peppers are tender.

7. Garnish with fresh cilantro before serving.

Nutrition Information:

- Calories: 280
- Protein: 12g
- Carbohydrates: 50g
- Fat: 4g
- Fiber: 12g
- Sugar: 7g
- Portion Size: 1 stuffed pepper

Greek Salad with Tofu Feta

Ingredients:

- 1 block (14 ounces) firm tofu, drained and pressed
- 2 tablespoons olive oil
- 2 tablespoons lemon juice
- 1 tablespoon apple cider vinegar
- 1 teaspoon dried oregano
- Salt and pepper to taste
- 2 cups cherry tomatoes, halved
- 1 cucumber, diced
- 1/2 red onion, thinly sliced
- 1/2 cup pitted Kalamata olives
- 1/4 cup chopped fresh parsley
- 1/4 cup crumbled vegan feta cheese (optional)

Instructions:

1. Cut the tofu into small cubes and place in a shallow dish.
2. In a small bowl, whisk together olive oil, lemon juice, apple cider vinegar, oregano, salt, and pepper.
3. Pour the dressing over the tofu cubes and toss to coat. Marinate for at least 30 minutes.

4. In a large bowl, combine marinated tofu, cherry tomatoes, cucumber, red onion, olives, and parsley.

5. Toss gently to combine.

6. Sprinkle with crumbled vegan feta cheese if desired before serving.

Nutrition Information:

- Calories: 220
- Protein: 12g
- Carbohydrates: 15g
- Fat: 14g
- Fiber: 5g
- Sugar: 6g
- Portion Size: 1 cup salad

Spinach and Mushroom Quesadillas

Ingredients:

- 4 large whole wheat tortillas
- 2 cups baby spinach leaves
- 1 cup sliced mushrooms
- 1/2 cup diced onion
- 1 clove garlic, minced

- 1 cup shredded vegan cheese

- 2 tablespoons olive oil

- Salt and pepper to taste

- Salsa and guacamole for serving

Instructions:

1. Heat 1 tablespoon of olive oil in a skillet over medium heat.

2. Add onion and garlic, and sauté until softened, about 2-3 minutes.

3. Add mushrooms and cook until they release their moisture and become tender, about 5 minutes.

4. Season with salt and pepper to taste.

5. Remove mushroom mixture from the skillet and set aside.

6. In the same skillet, add remaining olive oil and place one tortilla.

7. Layer spinach leaves, mushroom mixture, and shredded vegan cheese on one half of the tortilla.

8. Fold the tortilla in half to cover the filling.

9. Cook for 2-3 minutes on each side until golden brown and crispy.

10. Repeat with remaining tortillas and filling ingredients.

11. Cut quesadillas into wedges and serve with salsa and guacamole.

Nutrition Information:

- Calories: 320
- Protein: 10g
- Carbohydrates: 25g
- Fat: 20g
- Fiber: 5g
- Sugar: 3g
- Portion Size: 1 quesadilla

Cauliflower Rice Stir-Fry

Ingredients:

- 1 head cauliflower, grated into rice-like pieces
- 2 tablespoons soy sauce
- 1 tablespoon sesame oil
- 1 tablespoon rice vinegar
- 1 tablespoon maple syrup
- 1 tablespoon minced ginger

- 2 cloves garlic, minced
- 1 cup mixed vegetables (such as bell peppers, carrots, and peas)
- 1/4 cup chopped green onions
- Sesame seeds for garnish (optional)

Instructions:

1. In a small bowl, whisk together soy sauce, sesame oil, rice vinegar, and maple syrup to make the sauce.
2. Heat a large skillet over medium heat and add the minced ginger and garlic. Cook for 1 minute until fragrant.
3. Add the grated cauliflower and mixed vegetables to the skillet. Cook for 5-7 minutes until the vegetables are tender.
4. Pour the sauce over the cauliflower rice and vegetables. Stir to coat evenly.
5. Cook for an additional 2-3 minutes until everything is heated through.
6. Garnish with chopped green onions and sesame seeds before serving.

Nutrition Information:

- Calories: 150
- Protein: 5g
- Carbohydrates: 20g
- Fat: 7g
- Fiber: 7g
- Sugar: 9g
- Portion Size: 1 cup

Vegan Caesar Salad with Tempeh Bacon

Ingredients:

- 1 head romaine lettuce, chopped
- 1 cup cherry tomatoes, halved
- 1/4 cup vegan Caesar dressing
- 1/4 cup croutons
- 1/4 cup grated vegan parmesan cheese
- 1 package (8 ounces) tempeh, sliced thinly
- 2 tablespoons soy sauce
- 1 tablespoon maple syrup
- 1 tablespoon liquid smoke

- 1 tablespoon olive oil

Instructions:

1. Preheat the oven to 400°F (200°C).

2. In a small bowl, whisk together soy sauce, maple syrup, liquid smoke, and olive oil.

3. Place the sliced tempeh in a shallow dish and pour the marinade over it. Let it marinate for at least 15 minutes.

4. Place the marinated tempeh on a baking sheet lined with parchment paper. Bake for 15-20 minutes until crispy, flipping halfway through.

5. In a large bowl, combine chopped romaine lettuce, cherry tomatoes, vegan Caesar dressing, croutons, and grated vegan parmesan cheese.

6. Toss to coat evenly.

7. Top the salad with the crispy tempeh bacon before serving.

Nutrition Information:

- Calories: 280
- Protein: 12g

- Carbohydrates: 25g

- Fat: 15g

- Fiber: 7g

- Sugar: 6g

- Portion Size: 1.5 cups

Black Bean and Corn Tacos

Ingredients:

- 1 can (15 ounces) black beans, drained and rinsed

- 1 cup corn kernels

- 1 bell pepper, diced

- 1/2 onion, diced

- 2 cloves garlic, minced

- 1 teaspoon cumin

- 1 teaspoon chili powder

- Salt and pepper to taste

- 8 small corn tortillas

- Toppings: shredded lettuce, diced tomatoes, avocado slices, salsa, lime wedges

Instructions:

1. In a skillet over medium heat, sauté the diced onion and bell pepper until softened, about 5 minutes.
2. Add the minced garlic, cumin, chili powder, salt, and pepper. Cook for an additional minute until fragrant.
3. Stir in the black beans and corn kernels. Cook for 3-4 minutes until heated through.
4. Warm the corn tortillas in a separate skillet or in the microwave.
5. Spoon the black bean and corn mixture onto each tortilla.
6. Top with shredded lettuce, diced tomatoes, avocado slices, salsa, and a squeeze of lime juice.
7. Serve immediately.

Nutrition Information:

- Calories: 220
- Protein: 8g
- Carbohydrates: 40g
- Fat: 3g
- Fiber: 10g
- Sugar: 4g

- Portion Size: 2 tacos

Sweet Potato and Kale Buddha Bowl

Ingredients:

- 2 medium sweet potatoes, peeled and diced
- 2 cups kale, stems removed and chopped
- 1 can (15 ounces) chickpeas, drained and rinsed
- 1 tablespoon olive oil
- 1 teaspoon smoked paprika
- 1 teaspoon garlic powder
- Salt and pepper to taste
- Cooked quinoa or brown rice for serving
- Tahini dressing for drizzling

Instructions:

1. Preheat the oven to 400°F (200°C).
2. Toss the diced sweet potatoes with olive oil, smoked paprika, garlic powder, salt, and pepper.
3. Spread the sweet potatoes in a single layer on a baking sheet lined with parchment paper.
4. Roast in the preheated oven for 20-25 minutes until tender and slightly caramelized.

5. In a skillet over medium heat, sauté the chopped kale until wilted, about 3-4 minutes.

6. Add the chickpeas to the skillet and cook for an additional 2-3 minutes until heated through.

7. To assemble the Buddha bowls, divide cooked quinoa or brown rice among serving bowls.

8. Top with roasted sweet potatoes, sautéed kale, and chickpeas.

9. Drizzle with tahini dressing before serving.

Nutrition Information:

- Calories: 380
- Protein: 12g
- Carbohydrates: 60g
- Fat: 10g
- Fiber: 12g
- Sugar: 9g
- Portion Size: 1 bowl

Vegan BLT Sandwiches

Ingredients:

- 8 slices whole grain bread

- 1 cup vegan bacon strips or tempeh bacon

- 1 large tomato, sliced

- 1 cup lettuce leaves

- Vegan mayonnaise

- Mustard (optional)

- Salt and pepper to taste

Instructions:

1. Cook the vegan bacon strips or tempeh bacon according to package instructions until crispy.

2. Toast the whole grain bread slices until golden brown.

3. Spread vegan mayonnaise on one side of each bread slice.

4. Layer lettuce leaves on four bread slices.

5. Top with sliced tomato and crispy vegan bacon.

6. Season with salt and pepper to taste.

7. Optionally, spread mustard on the other four bread slices.

8. Place the mustard-side down on top of the bacon to form sandwiches.

9. Slice each sandwich in half diagonally and serve.

Nutrition Information:

- Calories: 280
- Protein: 10g
- Carbohydrates: 30g
- Fat: 14g
- Fiber: 6g
- Sugar: 4g
- Portion Size: 1 sandwich

Thai Peanut Noodle Salad

Ingredients:

- 8 ounces whole wheat spaghetti or rice noodles
- 1/4 cup creamy peanut butter
- 2 tablespoons soy sauce
- 2 tablespoons rice vinegar
- 1 tablespoon maple syrup
- 1 tablespoon lime juice
- 1 teaspoon minced ginger
- 2 cloves garlic, minced
- 1 bell pepper, thinly sliced
- 1 carrot, julienned
- 1/2 cucumber, thinly sliced

- 1/4 cup chopped peanuts
- Fresh cilantro for garnish

Instructions:

1. Cook the noodles according to package instructions until al dente. Drain and rinse under cold water to stop the cooking process.
2. In a small bowl, whisk together peanut butter, soy sauce, rice vinegar, maple syrup, lime juice, minced ginger, and minced garlic to make the dressing.
3. In a large bowl, combine cooked noodles, bell pepper, carrot, cucumber, and chopped peanuts.
4. Pour the peanut dressing over the noodle mixture and toss to coat evenly.
5. Garnish with fresh cilantro before serving.

Nutrition Information:

- Calories: 320
- Protein: 12g
- Carbohydrates: 45g
- Fat: 12g
- Fiber: 8g

- Sugar: 8g

- Portion Size: 1.5 cups

Mediterranean Veggie Wrap

Ingredients:

- 4 whole wheat wraps or tortillas

- 1 cup hummus

- 1 cup mixed greens

- 1/2 cucumber, sliced

- 1/2 bell pepper, thinly sliced

- 1/4 red onion, thinly sliced

- 1/4 cup sliced black olives

- 1/4 cup crumbled feta cheese (optional)

- Fresh parsley for garnish

Instructions:

1. Spread hummus evenly over each whole wheat wrap or tortilla.

2. Layer mixed greens, sliced cucumber, bell pepper, red onion, black olives, and crumbled feta cheese (if using) on each wrap.

3. Roll up the wraps tightly, tucking in the sides as you
    go.

4. Slice each wrap in half diagonally and secure with
    toothpicks if necessary.

5. Garnish with fresh parsley before serving.

Nutrition Information:

- Calories: 280

- Protein: 10g

- Carbohydrates: 35g

- Fat: 12g

- Fiber: 8g

- Sugar: 5g

- Portion Size: 1 wrap

Broccoli and White Bean Soup

Ingredients:

- 1 tablespoon olive oil

- 1 onion, chopped

- 2 cloves garlic, minced

- 4 cups vegetable broth

- 1 head broccoli, chopped

- 1 can (15 ounces) white beans, drained and rinsed
- 1 teaspoon dried thyme
- Salt and pepper to taste
- Fresh lemon juice for garnish
- Fresh parsley for garnish

Instructions:

1. Heat olive oil in a large pot over medium heat. Add chopped onion and garlic, and sauté until softened, about 5 minutes.
2. Add vegetable broth, chopped broccoli, white beans, dried thyme, salt, and pepper to the pot.
3. Bring the soup to a boil, then reduce heat and simmer for 15-20 minutes until the broccoli is tender.
4. Use an immersion blender to blend the soup until smooth. Alternatively, transfer the soup to a blender and blend in batches until smooth.
5. Adjust seasoning with additional salt and pepper if needed.
6. Ladle the soup into bowls, garnish with a squeeze of fresh lemon juice and chopped parsley, and serve hot.

Nutrition Information:

- Calories: 220
- Protein: 10g
- Carbohydrates: 30g
- Fat: 6g
- Fiber: 10g
- Sugar: 5g
- Portion Size: 1 cup

Edamame and Avocado Sushi Rolls

Ingredients:

- 2 cups cooked sushi rice
- 4 nori seaweed sheets
- 1 cup shelled edamame, cooked
- 1 ripe avocado, thinly sliced
- 1/2 cucumber, julienned
- 1 carrot, julienned
- Pickled ginger, for serving
- Soy sauce, for serving
- Wasabi, for serving

Instructions:

1. Place a nori seaweed sheet on a clean, dry surface.

2. Spread a thin layer of sushi rice evenly over the nori sheet, leaving about an inch of space at the top edge.

3. Arrange edamame, avocado slices, cucumber, and carrot in a line across the center of the rice.

4. Carefully roll up the sushi, using a bamboo sushi mat or your hands to tightly roll it.

5. Moisten the top edge of the nori sheet with water to seal the roll.

6. Repeat with the remaining nori sheets and filling ingredients.

7. Slice each sushi roll into bite-sized pieces using a sharp knife.

8. Serve with pickled ginger, soy sauce, and wasabi on the side.

Nutrition Information:

- Calories: 250
- Protein: 8g
- Carbohydrates: 40g
- Fat: 7g

- Fiber: 8g

- Sugar: 3g

- Portion Size: 1 roll

Mexican Quinoa Salad

Ingredients:

- 1 cup quinoa, cooked

- 1 can (15 ounces) black beans, drained and rinsed

- 1 cup corn kernels

- 1 bell pepper, diced

- 1/2 red onion, finely chopped

- 1 jalapeño, seeded and diced

- 1/4 cup chopped fresh cilantro

- 1 avocado, diced

- Juice of 2 limes

- 2 tablespoons olive oil

- 1 teaspoon cumin

- Salt and pepper to taste

- Tortilla chips for serving

Instructions:

1. In a large bowl, combine cooked quinoa, black beans, corn kernels, diced bell pepper, chopped red onion, diced jalapeño, and chopped fresh cilantro.

2. In a small bowl, whisk together lime juice, olive oil, cumin, salt, and pepper to make the dressing.

3. Pour the dressing over the quinoa mixture and toss to coat evenly.

4. Gently fold in diced avocado.

5. Serve the salad at room temperature or chilled, with tortilla chips on the side.

Nutrition Information:

- Calories: 320
- Protein: 10g
- Carbohydrates: 45g
- Fat: 12g
- Fiber: 12g
- Sugar: 5g
- Portion Size: 1.5 cups

Chapter 4: Dinner Recipes

These plant-based creations are not only bursting with flavor but are also crafted to help manage blood sugar levels effectively. From hearty classics like Vegan Shepherd's Pie to exotic dishes like Moroccan Chickpea Tagine, each recipe is a testament to the delicious possibilities of a plant-based diet.

Eggplant Parmesan with Whole Wheat Pasta

Ingredients:

- 1 large eggplant, sliced
- 1 cup whole wheat breadcrumbs
- 1 cup marinara sauce
- 1 cup vegan mozzarella cheese, shredded
- Fresh basil leaves, for garnish
- Salt and pepper to taste

Instructions:

1. Preheat the oven to 375°F (190°C).

2. Season eggplant slices with salt and pepper. Dip each slice in breadcrumbs, ensuring even coating.

3. Place eggplant slices on a baking sheet lined with parchment paper. Bake for 20-25 minutes until golden brown.

4. In a baking dish, spread a layer of marinara sauce. Arrange baked eggplant slices on top.

5. Sprinkle vegan mozzarella cheese over the eggplant. Repeat layers if desired.

6. Bake in the oven for another 15-20 minutes until the cheese is melted and bubbly.

7. Garnish with fresh basil leaves before serving.

Nutrition Information (per serving):

- Calories: 320
- Protein: 15g
- Carbohydrates: 45g
- Fat: 10g
- Fiber: 12g
- Sugar: 8g
- Portion Size: 1 serving

Vegan Chili with Beans and Sweet Potatoes

Ingredients:

- 2 cups cooked black beans
- 1 cup cooked kidney beans
- 1 onion, diced
- 2 cloves garlic, minced
- 2 sweet potatoes, diced
- 1 can diced tomatoes
- 1 cup vegetable broth
- 1 tablespoon chili powder
- 1 teaspoon cumin
- Salt and pepper to taste

Instructions:

1. In a large pot, sauté onion and garlic until fragrant.
2. Add diced sweet potatoes and cook for 5 minutes.
3. Stir in diced tomatoes, vegetable broth, chili powder, and cumin.
4. Bring to a simmer and let it cook for 20-25 minutes until sweet potatoes are tender.

5. Add cooked black beans and kidney beans to the pot. Cook for an additional 10 minutes.

6. Season with salt and pepper to taste before serving.

Nutrition Information (per serving):

- Calories: 280
- Protein: 10g
- Carbohydrates: 50g
- Fat: 2g
- Fiber: 15g
- Sugar: 10g
- Portion Size: 1 serving

Stuffed Portobello Mushrooms

Ingredients:

- 4 large portobello mushrooms
- 1 cup quinoa, cooked
- 1 cup spinach, chopped
- 1/2 cup cherry tomatoes, halved
- 1/4 cup vegan parmesan cheese, grated
- 2 cloves garlic, minced
- 1 tablespoon balsamic vinegar

- Salt and pepper to taste

Instructions:

1. Preheat the oven to 375°F (190°C). Remove stems from portobello mushrooms and gently scrape out gills.
2. In a bowl, mix cooked quinoa, chopped spinach, halved cherry tomatoes, vegan parmesan cheese, minced garlic, and balsamic vinegar. Season with salt and pepper.
3. Stuff each portobello mushroom with the quinoa mixture.
4. Place stuffed mushrooms on a baking sheet lined with parchment paper. Bake for 20-25 minutes until mushrooms are tender.
5. Serve hot, garnished with additional vegan parmesan cheese if desired.

Nutrition Information (per serving):

- Calories: 200
- Protein: 10g
- Carbohydrates: 30g

- Fat: 5g

- Fiber: 5g

- Sugar: 5g

- Portion Size: 1 serving

Ratatouille with Quinoa

Ingredients:

- 1 eggplant, diced

- 2 zucchinis, diced

- 1 yellow bell pepper, diced

- 1 red onion, diced

- 2 cloves garlic, minced

- 1 can diced tomatoes

- 1 teaspoon dried thyme

- 1 teaspoon dried oregano

- Salt and pepper to taste

- 1 cup cooked quinoa

Instructions:

1. In a large skillet, sauté diced eggplant, zucchinis, yellow bell pepper, red onion, and minced garlic until vegetables are tender.

2. Stir in diced tomatoes, dried thyme, and dried oregano. Season with salt and pepper.

3. Let the mixture simmer for 15-20 minutes until flavors meld together.

4. Serve ratatouille over cooked quinoa.

Nutrition Information (per serving):

- Calories: 250
- Protein: 8g
- Carbohydrates: 45g
- Fat: 3g
- Fiber: 10g
- Sugar: 10g
- Portion Size: 1 serving

Cauliflower Curry with Brown Rice

Ingredients:

- 1 small cauliflower, cut into florets
- 1 onion, diced
- 2 cloves garlic, minced
- 1 can coconut milk
- 2 tablespoons curry powder

- 1 teaspoon turmeric powder
- 1 teaspoon cumin
- Salt and pepper to taste
- 2 cups cooked brown rice

Instructions:

1. In a large skillet, sauté diced onion and minced garlic until softened.
2. Add cauliflower florets to the skillet and cook until slightly browned.
3. Stir in coconut milk, curry powder, turmeric powder, and cumin. Season with salt and pepper.
4. Let the mixture simmer for 15-20 minutes until cauliflower is tender and the sauce thickens.
5. Serve cauliflower curry over cooked brown rice.

Nutrition Information (per serving):

- Calories: 300
- Protein: 7g
- Carbohydrates: 45g
- Fat: 10g
- Fiber: 8g

- Sugar: 5g

- Portion Size: 1 serving

Spaghetti Squash Primavera

Ingredients:

- 1 large spaghetti squash

- 2 cups mixed vegetables (bell peppers, broccoli, cherry tomatoes, etc.), diced

- 2 cloves garlic, minced

- 1/4 cup vegetable broth

- 1 tablespoon olive oil

- 1 teaspoon Italian seasoning

- Salt and pepper to taste

Instructions:

1. Preheat the oven to 375°F (190°C). Cut spaghetti squash in half lengthwise and remove seeds.

2. Place spaghetti squash halves cut-side down on a baking sheet lined with parchment paper. Bake for 30-40 minutes until tender.

3. Meanwhile, in a skillet, sauté mixed vegetables and minced garlic in olive oil until vegetables are tender.

4. Add vegetable broth and Italian seasoning to the skillet. Season with salt and pepper.

5. Using a fork, scrape the flesh of the cooked spaghetti squash into "noodles."

6. Serve spaghetti squash noodles topped with primavera sauce.

Nutrition Information (per serving):

- Calories: 220
- Protein: 5g
- Carbohydrates: 35g
- Fat: 8g
- Fiber: 10g
- Sugar: 10g
- Portion Size: 1 serving

Vegan Shepherd's Pie

Ingredients:

- 4 large potatoes, peeled and diced
- 1 cup green lentils, cooked
- 1 onion, diced
- 2 carrots, diced

- 1 cup peas, fresh or frozen

- 2 cloves garlic, minced

- 1 cup vegetable broth

- 2 tablespoons tomato paste

- 1 teaspoon thyme

- Salt and pepper to taste

Instructions:

1. Preheat the oven to 375°F (190°C). Boil diced potatoes until tender, then mash them with a fork or potato masher.

2. In a skillet, sauté diced onion, carrots, and minced garlic until softened.

3. Stir in cooked green lentils, peas, vegetable broth, tomato paste, and thyme. Season with salt and pepper.

4. Let the mixture simmer for 10-15 minutes until flavors meld together.

5. Transfer the lentil mixture into a baking dish and spread mashed potatoes on top.

6. Bake in the oven for 25-30 minutes until the top is golden brown.

7. Serve hot and enjoy!

Nutrition Information (per serving):

- Calories: 280
- Protein: 10g
- Carbohydrates: 50g
- Fat: 3g
- Fiber: 12g
- Sugar: 8g
- Portion Size: 1 serving

Lentil Sloppy Joes

Ingredients:

- 1 cup green lentils, cooked
- 1 onion, diced
- 2 cloves garlic, minced
- 1 bell pepper, diced
- 1 can crushed tomatoes
- 2 tablespoons tomato paste
- 1 tablespoon maple syrup
- 1 tablespoon apple cider vinegar
- 1 teaspoon chili powder

- Salt and pepper to taste
- Whole grain burger buns

Instructions:

1. In a skillet, sauté diced onion, minced garlic, and diced bell pepper until softened.
2. Stir in cooked green lentils, crushed tomatoes, tomato paste, maple syrup, apple cider vinegar, and chili powder.
3. Let the mixture simmer for 15-20 minutes until thickened.
4. Season with salt and pepper to taste.
5. Serve lentil sloppy joe mixture on whole grain burger buns.

Nutrition Information (per serving):

- Calories: 250
- Protein: 12g
- Carbohydrates: 45g
- Fat: 2g
- Fiber: 10g
- Sugar: 10g

- Portion Size: 1 serving

Mushroom and Spinach Vegan Lasagna

Ingredients:

- 9 lasagna noodles, cooked according to package instructions
- 2 cups mushrooms, sliced
- 2 cups spinach
- 2 cloves garlic, minced
- 1 onion, diced
- 2 cups marinara sauce
- 1 cup vegan ricotta cheese
- 1 cup vegan mozzarella cheese, shredded
- Salt and pepper to taste

Instructions:

1. Preheat the oven to 375°F (190°C). In a skillet, sauté diced onion and minced garlic until fragrant.

2. Add sliced mushrooms and cook until tender. Stir in spinach and cook until wilted. Season with salt and pepper.

3. In a baking dish, spread a layer of marinara sauce. Place three cooked lasagna noodles on top.

4. Spread half of the mushroom and spinach mixture over the noodles. Dollop half of the vegan ricotta cheese on top.

5. Repeat layers with marinara sauce, lasagna noodles, remaining mushroom and spinach mixture, and vegan ricotta cheese.

6. Finish with a final layer of marinara sauce and sprinkle vegan mozzarella cheese on top.

7. Cover the baking dish with aluminum foil and bake for 30 minutes.

8. Remove the foil and bake for an additional 10-15 minutes until the cheese is melted and bubbly.

9. Let the lasagna cool for a few minutes before slicing and serving.

Nutrition Information (per serving):
- Calories: 320

- Protein: 15g

- Carbohydrates: 40g

- Fat: 10g

- Fiber: 8g

- Sugar: 10g

- Portion Size: 1 serving

Teriyaki Tofu Stir-Fry

Ingredients:

- 1 block tofu, pressed and cubed

- 2 cups mixed vegetables (bell peppers, broccoli, snap peas, carrots, etc.)

- 1/4 cup teriyaki sauce

- 2 tablespoons soy sauce

- 1 tablespoon sesame oil

- 2 cloves garlic, minced

- 1 teaspoon ginger, minced

- Cooked brown rice for serving

Instructions:

1. In a large skillet or wok, heat sesame oil over medium heat. Add minced garlic and ginger, and sauté until fragrant.
2. Add cubed tofu to the skillet and cook until golden brown on all sides.
3. Stir in mixed vegetables and cook until tender-crisp.
4. Pour teriyaki sauce and soy sauce over the tofu and vegetables. Stir to coat evenly.
5. Let the stir-fry simmer for a few minutes until the sauce thickens slightly.
6. Serve hot over cooked brown rice.

Nutrition Information (per serving):

- Calories: 300
- Protein: 20g
- Carbohydrates: 35g
- Fat: 10g
- Fiber: 8g
- Sugar: 10g
- Portion Size: 1 serving

Butternut Squash Risotto

Ingredients:

- 2 cups butternut squash, diced
- 1 onion, diced
- 2 cloves garlic, minced
- 1 cup Arborio rice
- 4 cups vegetable broth, warmed
- 1/4 cup nutritional yeast
- 2 tablespoons olive oil
- Salt and pepper to taste
- Fresh parsley, chopped, for garnish

Instructions:

1. In a large skillet, heat olive oil over medium heat. Add diced onion and minced garlic, sauté until softened.

2. Add Arborio rice to the skillet and toast for 2-3 minutes until lightly golden.

3. Gradually add warm vegetable broth, 1/2 cup at a time, stirring constantly and allowing the liquid to absorb before adding more.

4. When the rice is almost cooked, stir in diced butternut squash and continue cooking until the squash is tender and the rice is creamy.

5. Stir in nutritional yeast and season with salt and pepper to taste.

6. Garnish with fresh chopped parsley before serving.

Nutrition Information (per serving):

- Calories: 280
- Protein: 6g
- Carbohydrates: 50g
- Fat: 6g
- Fiber: 8g
- Sugar: 5g
- Portion Size: 1 serving

Black Bean Enchiladas

Ingredients:

- 1 can black beans, drained and rinsed
- 1 onion, diced
- 1 bell pepper, diced
- 1 cup corn kernels

- 1 cup enchilada sauce

- 1 cup vegan cheese, shredded

- 8 whole wheat tortillas

- Fresh cilantro, chopped, for garnish

Instructions:

1. Preheat the oven to 375°F (190°C). In a skillet, sauté diced onion and bell pepper until softened.

2. Stir in black beans and corn kernels, cook for a few minutes until heated through.

3. Spread a thin layer of enchilada sauce on the bottom of a baking dish.

4. Place a spoonful of the black bean mixture in the center of each tortilla, roll up tightly, and place seam-side down in the baking dish.

5. Pour remaining enchilada sauce over the rolled tortillas, then sprinkle vegan cheese on top.

6. Bake in the oven for 20-25 minutes until the cheese is melted and bubbly.

7. Garnish with fresh chopped cilantro before serving.

Nutrition Information (per serving):

- Calories: 320
- Protein: 12g
- Carbohydrates: 45g
- Fat: 8g
- Fiber: 10g
- Sugar: 5g
- Portion Size: 1 serving

Moroccan Chickpea Tagine

Ingredients:

- 2 cups cooked chickpeas
- 1 onion, diced
- 2 cloves garlic, minced
- 1 bell pepper, diced
- 1 carrot, diced
- 1 can diced tomatoes
- 1 cup vegetable broth
- 1/2 cup dried apricots, chopped
- 1 teaspoon ground cumin
- 1 teaspoon ground coriander
- 1/2 teaspoon ground cinnamon

- Salt and pepper to taste
- Fresh parsley, chopped, for garnish
- Cooked couscous or quinoa for serving

Instructions:

1. In a large pot or tagine, sauté diced onion and minced garlic until fragrant.
2. Add diced bell pepper and carrot, cook until softened.
3. Stir in cooked chickpeas, diced tomatoes, vegetable broth, chopped dried apricots, ground cumin, ground coriander, and ground cinnamon.
4. Season with salt and pepper to taste. Cover and let simmer for 20-25 minutes to allow flavors to meld together.
5. Serve hot over cooked couscous or quinoa.
6. Garnish with fresh chopped parsley before serving.

Nutrition Information (per serving):

- Calories: 280
- Protein: 10g
- Carbohydrates: 50g

- Fat: 3g

- Fiber: 12g

- Sugar: 10g

- Portion Size: 1 serving

Coconut Curry Lentil Soup

Ingredients:

- 1 cup red lentils
- 1 onion, diced
- 2 cloves garlic, minced
- 1 bell pepper, diced
- 1 carrot, diced
- 1 can coconut milk
- 4 cups vegetable broth
- 2 tablespoons curry powder
- 1 teaspoon turmeric
- Salt and pepper to taste
- Fresh cilantro, chopped, for garnish

Instructions:

1. In a large pot, sauté diced onion and minced garlic
   until fragrant.

2. Add diced bell pepper and carrot, cook until softened.

3. Rinse red lentils under cold water, then add to the pot along with coconut milk, vegetable broth, curry powder, and turmeric.

4. Bring to a boil, then reduce heat and let simmer for 20-25 minutes until lentils are cooked and soup has thickened.

5. Season with salt and pepper to taste.

6. Serve hot, garnished with fresh chopped cilantro.

Nutrition Information (per serving):

- Calories: 300
- Protein: 15g
- Carbohydrates: 40g
- Fat: 10g
- Fiber: 8g
- Sugar: 5g
- Portion Size: 1 serving

Vegan Pad Thai

Ingredients:

- 8 oz rice noodles
- 1 block tofu, pressed and cubed
- 2 tablespoons soy sauce
- 2 tablespoons lime juice
- 2 tablespoons maple syrup
- 2 cloves garlic, minced
- 1 red bell pepper, sliced
- 1 carrot, julienned
- 1 cup bean sprouts
- 2 green onions, chopped
- Crushed peanuts and fresh cilantro, for garnish

Instructions:

1. Cook rice noodles according to package instructions, then drain and set aside.
2. In a skillet, sauté cubed tofu in soy sauce until lightly browned.
3. Add minced garlic, sliced red bell pepper, and julienned carrot to the skillet. Cook until vegetables are tender.

4. Stir in cooked rice noodles, lime juice, maple syrup, bean sprouts, and chopped green onions. Toss to combine.

5. Cook for a few minutes until heated through.

6. Serve hot, garnished with crushed peanuts and fresh cilantro.

Nutrition Information (per serving):

- Calories: 320
- Protein: 12g
- Carbohydrates: 50g
- Fat: 8g
- Fiber: 5g
- Sugar: 10g
- Portion Size: 1 serving

Chapter 5: Snacks and Appetizers

In this chapter, we present delectable plant-based options that not only satisfy cravings but also provide essential nutrients to support your health goals. From crunchy kale chips to savory stuffed mini bell peppers, these recipes are bursting with flavor and goodness. Enjoy these snacks guilt-free while nourishing your body with every bite.

Hummus and Veggie Sticks

Ingredients:

- 1 cup chickpeas (cooked or canned)
- 2 tablespoons tahini
- 2 tablespoons lemon juice
- 1 clove garlic, minced
- 2 tablespoons olive oil
- Salt and pepper to taste
- Assorted vegetable sticks (carrots, celery, bell peppers)

Instructions:

1. In a food processor, blend the chickpeas, tahini, lemon juice, garlic, and olive oil until smooth.
2. Season with salt and pepper to taste.
3. Serve the hummus with assorted vegetable sticks for dipping.

Nutrition Information (per serving):

*   Calories: 120
*   Protein: 4g
*   Carbohydrates: 12g
*   Fat: 7g
*   Fiber: 4g
*   Sugar: 2g
*   Portion size: 2 tablespoons of hummus with vegetable sticks

Guacamole with Baked Tortilla Chips

Ingredients:

*   2 ripe avocados

- 1 tomato, diced
- 1/4 cup onion, finely chopped
- 1/4 cup cilantro, chopped
- 1 lime, juiced
- Salt and pepper to taste
- Whole grain tortillas

Instructions:

1. In a bowl, mash the avocados until smooth.
2. Stir in the diced tomato, chopped onion, chopped cilantro, and lime juice.
3. Season with salt and pepper to taste.
4. Cut the whole grain tortillas into wedges and bake in the oven until crisp.
5. Serve the guacamole with the baked tortilla chips.

Nutrition Information (per serving):

- Calories: 160
- Protein: 3g
- Carbohydrates: 20g
- Fat: 9g
- Fiber: 7g

- Sugar: 2g
- Portion size: 1/4 cup guacamole with baked tortilla chips

Roasted Chickpeas

Ingredients:

- 1 can chickpeas, drained and rinsed
- 1 tablespoon olive oil
- 1 teaspoon paprika
- 1 teaspoon garlic powder
- Salt to taste

Instructions:

1. Preheat the oven to 400°F (200°C).
2. In a bowl, toss the chickpeas with olive oil, paprika, garlic powder, and salt until evenly coated.
3. Spread the chickpeas in a single layer on a baking sheet.
4. Roast in the preheated oven for 25-30 minutes, stirring occasionally, until crispy.
5. Let cool before serving.

Nutrition Information (per serving):

- Calories: 140
- Protein: 6g
- Carbohydrates: 20g
- Fat: 4g
- Fiber: 6g
- Sugar: 4g
- Portion size: 1/2 cup roasted chickpeas

Sliced Apple with Almond Butter

Ingredients:

- 1 medium apple, sliced
- 2 tablespoons almond butter

Instructions:

1. Slice the apple into wedges or rounds.
2. Spread almond butter on each apple slice.
3. Arrange on a plate and serve.

Nutrition Information (per serving):

- Calories: 180
- Protein: 4g

- Carbohydrates: 20g

- Fat: 10g

- Fiber: 5g

- Sugar: 14g

- Portion size: 1 medium apple with 2 tablespoons almond butter

Trail Mix with Nuts and Seeds

Ingredients:

- 1/4 cup almonds

- 1/4 cup cashews

- 1/4 cup pumpkin seeds

- 1/4 cup dried cranberries

- 1/4 cup dark chocolate chips

Instructions:

1. In a bowl, mix together almonds, cashews, pumpkin seeds, dried cranberries, and dark chocolate chips.

2. Portion into small snack bags or containers for easy grab-and-go snacks.

Nutrition Information (per serving):

- Calories: 200
- Protein: 6g
- Carbohydrates: 15g
- Fat: 14g
- Fiber: 3g
- Sugar: 9g
- Portion size: 1/4 cup trail mix

Cucumber and Tomato Bruschetta

Ingredients:

- 1 cucumber, diced
- 1 tomato, diced
- 2 tablespoons red onion, finely chopped
- 2 tablespoons fresh basil, chopped
- 1 tablespoon balsamic vinegar
- 1 tablespoon olive oil
- Salt and pepper to taste
- Whole grain baguette slices, toasted (optional)

Instructions:

1. In a bowl, combine diced cucumber, tomato, red onion, and basil.
2. Drizzle with balsamic vinegar and olive oil.
3. Season with salt and pepper to taste.
4. Serve the bruschetta on toasted whole grain baguette slices if desired.

Nutrition Information (per serving):

- Calories: 90
- Protein: 2g
- Carbohydrates: 10g
- Fat: 5g
- Fiber: 2g
- Sugar: 4g
- Portion size: 1/2 cup bruschetta mixture

Veggie Sushi Rolls

Ingredients:

- Nori seaweed sheets
- Cooked sushi rice

- Assorted vegetables (cucumber, avocado, carrot, bell pepper, etc.)
- Soy sauce or tamari, for dipping
- Pickled ginger and wasabi, optional

Instructions:

1. Place a nori sheet on a bamboo sushi mat or flat surface.
2. Spread a thin layer of sushi rice over the nori, leaving a 1-inch border at the top edge.
3. Arrange thinly sliced vegetables in the center of the rice.
4. Roll the nori tightly around the vegetables, using the bamboo mat to help shape the roll.
5. Slice the sushi roll into bite-sized pieces using a sharp knife.
6. Serve with soy sauce, pickled ginger, and wasabi if desired.

Nutrition Information (per serving):
- Calories: 120
- Protein: 3g

- Carbohydrates: 25g

- Fat: 1g

- Fiber: 3g

- Sugar: 1g

- Portion size: 6 sushi pieces

Kale Chips

Ingredients:

- 1 bunch kale, stems removed and leaves torn into bite-sized pieces

- 1 tablespoon olive oil

- Salt and pepper to taste

Instructions:

1. Preheat the oven to 300°F (150°C).

2. In a large bowl, toss kale leaves with olive oil, salt, and pepper until evenly coated.

3. Spread the kale in a single layer on a baking sheet.

4. Bake in the preheated oven for 10-15 minutes, or until crispy.

5. Let cool before serving.

Nutrition Information (per serving):

- Calories: 50
- Protein: 2g
- Carbohydrates: 5g
- Fat: 3g
- Fiber: 2g
- Sugar: 1g
- Portion size: 1 cup kale chips

Stuffed Mini Bell Peppers

Ingredients:

- Mini bell peppers
- Hummus or vegan cream cheese
- Assorted fillings (cucumber, carrot, avocado, sprouts, etc.)

Instructions:

1. Cut the tops off the mini bell peppers and remove the seeds.
2. Fill each pepper with hummus or vegan cream cheese.
3. Add assorted fillings to each pepper.

4. Serve chilled or at room temperature.

Nutrition Information (per serving):

- Calories: 40

- Protein: 1g

- Carbohydrates: 5g

- Fat: 2g

- Fiber: 1g

- Sugar: 2g

- Portion size: 3 stuffed mini bell peppers

Spicy Edamame

Ingredients:

- 2 cups edamame (shelled)

- 1 tablespoon sesame oil

- 1 teaspoon chili powder

- 1/2 teaspoon garlic powder

- Salt to taste

Instructions:

1. Boil the shelled edamame in salted water for 3-4 minutes, then drain.

2. In a skillet, heat sesame oil over medium heat.

3. Add the boiled edamame to the skillet and sauté for 2-3 minutes.

4. Sprinkle chili powder, garlic powder, and salt over the edamame, stirring to coat evenly.

5. Cook for an additional 2-3 minutes, until heated through.

6. Serve hot or cold.

Nutrition Information (per serving):

- Calories: 120

- Protein: 9g

- Carbohydrates: 8g

- Fat: 5g

- Fiber: 4g

- Sugar: 2g

- Portion size: 1/2 cup spicy edamame

Vegan Cheese and Crackers

Ingredients:

- Vegan cheese slices or spread

- Whole grain crackers

- Assorted toppings (grape tomatoes, olives, cucumber slices, etc.)

Instructions:

1. Arrange vegan cheese slices or spread on a serving platter.
2. Place whole grain crackers alongside the cheese.
3. Add assorted toppings to the platter for variety.
4. Serve as a simple and satisfying snack.

Nutrition Information (per serving):

- Calories: 160
- Protein: 4g
- Carbohydrates: 20g
- Fat: 8g
- Fiber: 3g
- Sugar: 2g
- Portion size: 2 vegan cheese slices with 5 crackers

Avocado Cucumber Rolls

Ingredients:

- 1 ripe avocado, mashed

- 1 cucumber, peeled into thin strips

- 2 tablespoons hummus

- Whole grain tortillas or nori sheets

Instructions:

1. Lay a tortilla or nori sheet flat on a cutting board.

2. Spread a thin layer of mashed avocado and hummus over the surface.

3. Place cucumber strips along one edge of the tortilla or nori sheet.

4. Roll tightly into a cylinder shape, then slice into bite-sized pieces.

5. Secure with toothpicks if needed.

6. Serve chilled.

Nutrition Information (per serving):

- Calories: 110

- Protein: 3g

- Carbohydrates: 15g

- Fat: 6g

- Fiber: 5g

- Sugar: 2g

- Portion size: 6 avocado cucumber rolls

Mediterranean Stuffed Grape Leaves

Ingredients:

- 1 jar grape leaves, drained
- 1 cup cooked quinoa
- 1/4 cup chopped fresh parsley
- 1/4 cup chopped fresh mint
- 1/4 cup chopped sun-dried tomatoes
- 2 tablespoons pine nuts
- 2 tablespoons lemon juice
- Salt and pepper to taste

Instructions:

1. In a bowl, mix together cooked quinoa, chopped parsley, chopped mint, sun-dried tomatoes, pine nuts, lemon juice, salt, and pepper.
2. Lay a grape leaf flat on a clean surface.
3. Place a spoonful of the quinoa mixture in the center of the leaf.
4. Fold the sides of the leaf over the filling, then roll tightly into a cylinder shape.

5. Repeat with remaining grape leaves and filling.

6. Serve chilled or at room temperature.

Nutrition Information (per serving):

- Calories: 90

- Protein: 3g

- Carbohydrates: 15g

- Fat: 2g

- Fiber: 3g

- Sugar: 2g

- Portion size: 3 stuffed grape leaves

Sweet Potato Fries with Spicy Dipping Sauce

Ingredients for Sweet Potato Fries:

- 2 large sweet potatoes, cut into fries

- 1 tablespoon olive oil

- 1 teaspoon paprika

- 1/2 teaspoon garlic powder

- Salt and pepper to taste

Ingredients for Spicy Dipping Sauce:

- 1/4 cup vegan mayonnaise
- 1 tablespoon sriracha sauce
- 1 teaspoon lemon juice
- Pinch of salt

Instructions:

1. Preheat the oven to 425°F (220°C).
2. In a bowl, toss sweet potato fries with olive oil, paprika, garlic powder, salt, and pepper until evenly coated.
3. Spread the fries in a single layer on a baking sheet.
4. Bake in the preheated oven for 20-25 minutes, flipping halfway through, until crispy.
5. Meanwhile, mix together vegan mayonnaise, sriracha sauce, lemon juice, and salt to make the spicy dipping sauce.
6. Serve the sweet potato fries hot with the spicy dipping sauce on the side.

Nutrition Information (per serving):

- Calories: 180 (for sweet potato fries)

- Protein: 2g

- Carbohydrates: 30g

- Fat: 6g

- Fiber: 5g

- Sugar: 7g

- Portion size: 1 cup sweet potato fries with 2 tablespoons dipping sauce

Baked Tofu Bites

Ingredients:

- 1 block extra-firm tofu, pressed and cubed

- 2 tablespoons soy sauce or tamari

- 1 tablespoon maple syrup

- 1 teaspoon sesame oil

- 1/2 teaspoon garlic powder

- 1/2 teaspoon smoked paprika

- 1/4 teaspoon black pepper

Instructions:

1. Preheat the oven to 400°F (200°C) and line a baking sheet with parchment paper.

2. In a bowl, whisk together soy sauce, maple syrup, sesame oil, garlic powder, smoked paprika, and black pepper.

3. Add the cubed tofu to the bowl and toss to coat evenly.

4. Arrange the tofu cubes in a single layer on the prepared baking sheet.

5. Bake in the preheated oven for 25-30 minutes, flipping halfway through, until golden and crispy.

6. Serve hot or at room temperature.

Nutrition Information (per serving):

- Calories: 120
- Protein: 8g
- Carbohydrates: 8g
- Fat: 5g
- Fiber: 2g
- Sugar: 3g
- Portion size: 1/2 cup baked tofu cubes

Chapter 6: Desserts

Indulging in delicious desserts while managing blood sugar levels can be a challenge, but with these plant-based recipes, you can satisfy your sweet tooth without worrying about spikes in glucose levels. From creamy mousses to fruity popsicles, these desserts are not only tasty but also packed with nutrients to support your health journey.

Vegan Chocolate Avocado Mousse

Ingredients:

- 2 ripe avocados
- 1/4 cup cocoa powder
- 1/4 cup maple syrup
- 1 teaspoon vanilla extract
- Pinch of salt

Instructions:

1. Scoop the flesh of the avocados into a blender or food processor.

2. Add cocoa powder, maple syrup, vanilla extract, and salt.

3. Blend until smooth and creamy, scraping down the sides as needed.

4. Transfer the mousse into serving cups and chill in the refrigerator for at least 30 minutes before serving.

Nutrition Information (per serving):

- Calories: 180
- Protein: 2g
- Carbohydrates: 16g
- Fat: 12g
- Fiber: 6g
- Sugar: 8g
- Portion Size: 1/2 cup

Berry and Banana Nice Cream

Ingredients:

- 2 ripe bananas, sliced and frozen
- 1 cup mixed berries, frozen
- 1/4 cup almond milk (or any plant-based milk)

Instructions:

1. Place the frozen bananas, mixed berries, and almond milk in a blender or food processor.
2. Blend until smooth and creamy, scraping down the sides as needed.
3. Serve immediately as soft-serve ice cream or transfer to a container and freeze for a firmer texture.

Nutrition Information (per serving):

- Calories: 120
- Protein: 2g
- Carbohydrates: 28g
- Fat: 1g
- Fiber: 5g
- Sugar: 15g
- Portion Size: 1/2 cup

Pumpkin Spice Energy Bites

Ingredients:

- 1 cup rolled oats
- 1/2 cup pumpkin puree
- 1/4 cup almond butter

- 2 tablespoons maple syrup

- 1 teaspoon pumpkin pie spice

- 1/4 cup chopped nuts (such as walnuts or pecans)

Instructions:

1. In a mixing bowl, combine rolled oats, pumpkin puree, almond butter, maple syrup, and pumpkin pie spice.

2. Stir until well combined, then fold in chopped nuts.

3. Roll the mixture into small balls using your hands.

4. Place the energy bites on a baking sheet lined with parchment paper and refrigerate for at least 30 minutes before serving.

Nutrition Information (per serving):

- Calories: 90

- Protein: 3g

- Carbohydrates: 10g

- Fat: 5g

- Fiber: 2g

- Sugar: 3g

- Portion Size: 1 energy bite

Coconut Almond Macaroons

Ingredients:

- 2 cups shredded coconut (unsweetened)
- 1/2 cup almond flour
- 1/4 cup maple syrup
- 2 tablespoons coconut oil, melted
- 1 teaspoon vanilla extract
- Pinch of salt

Instructions:

1. Preheat the oven to 350°F (175°C). Line a baking sheet with parchment paper.
2. In a mixing bowl, combine shredded coconut, almond flour, maple syrup, melted coconut oil, vanilla extract, and salt. Mix well.
3. Scoop tablespoon-sized portions of the mixture onto the prepared baking sheet, shaping them into small mounds.
4. Bake for 12-15 minutes, or until the macaroons are golden brown around the edges.
5. Allow the macaroons to cool completely before serving.

Nutrition Information (per serving):

- Calories: 90
- Protein: 1g
- Carbohydrates: 7g
- Fat: 7g
- Fiber: 2g
- Sugar: 4g
- Portion Size: 1 macaroon

Chia Seed Berry Popsicles

Ingredients:

- 1 cup mixed berries (such as strawberries, blueberries, and raspberries)
- 2 tablespoons chia seeds
- 1 tablespoon maple syrup (optional)
- 1 1/2 cups coconut water or almond milk

Instructions:

1. In a blender, combine mixed berries, chia seeds, maple syrup (if using), and coconut water or almond milk.
2. Blend until smooth.

3. Pour the mixture into popsicle molds.

4. Insert popsicle sticks and freeze for at least 4 hours, or until solid.

5. Run the molds under warm water to release the popsicles before serving.

Nutrition Information (per serving):

- Calories: 40
- Protein: 1g
- Carbohydrates: 6g
- Fat: 2g
- Fiber: 3g
- Sugar: 3g
- Portion Size: 1 popsicle

Apple Cinnamon Oat Bars

Ingredients:

- 2 cups rolled oats
- 1 cup unsweetened applesauce
- 1/4 cup maple syrup
- 1 teaspoon cinnamon
- 1/4 cup chopped walnuts or almonds (optional)

Instructions:

1. Preheat the oven to 350°F (175°C). Grease a baking dish or line it with parchment paper.
2. In a mixing bowl, combine rolled oats, applesauce, maple syrup, cinnamon, and chopped nuts (if using).
3. Press the mixture into the prepared baking dish, spreading it out evenly.
4. Bake for 25-30 minutes, or until the edges are golden brown.
5. Allow the oat bars to cool completely before cutting into squares or bars.

Nutrition Information (per serving):

- Calories: 120
- Protein: 3g
- Carbohydrates: 21g
- Fat: 3g
- Fiber: 3g
- Sugar: 8g
- Portion Size: 1 bar

Vegan Peanut Butter Cups

Ingredients:

- 1/2 cup natural peanut butter
- 2 tablespoons maple syrup
- 1/4 cup coconut oil, melted
- 1/4 cup cocoa powder
- 1/4 teaspoon vanilla extract
- Pinch of salt

Instructions:

1. In a mixing bowl, combine peanut butter and maple syrup.
2. In a separate bowl, mix melted coconut oil, cocoa powder, vanilla extract, and salt until smooth.
3. Line a mini muffin tin with paper liners.
4. Spoon a small amount of the chocolate mixture into each liner, spreading it to cover the bottom.
5. Place a dollop of peanut butter mixture on top of the chocolate layer.
6. Cover the peanut butter with another layer of chocolate.
7. Freeze for about 30 minutes, or until set.

8. Store in the refrigerator until ready to serve.

Nutrition Information (per serving):

- Calories: 90
- Protein: 2g
- Carbohydrates: 6g
- Fat: 7g
- Fiber: 2g
- Sugar: 3g
- Portion Size: 1 peanut butter cup

Lemon Poppy Seed Muffins

Ingredients:

- 2 cups almond flour
- 1/4 cup coconut flour
- 1/4 cup maple syrup
- 1/4 cup lemon juice
- Zest of 1 lemon
- 2 tablespoons poppy seeds
- 1/2 teaspoon baking soda
- Pinch of salt
- 1/4 cup almond milk

- 1/4 cup coconut oil, melted
- 1 teaspoon vanilla extract

Instructions:

1. Preheat the oven to 350°F (175°C). Line a muffin tin with paper liners.
2. In a mixing bowl, combine almond flour, coconut flour, maple syrup, lemon juice, lemon zest, poppy seeds, baking soda, and salt.
3. In a separate bowl, whisk together almond milk, melted coconut oil, and vanilla extract.
4. Pour the wet ingredients into the dry ingredients and stir until well combined.
5. Divide the batter evenly among the muffin cups.
6. Bake for 20-25 minutes, or until a toothpick inserted into the center comes out clean.
7. Allow the muffins to cool in the tin for 5 minutes before transferring to a wire rack to cool completely.

Nutrition Information (per serving):

- Calories: 180
- Protein: 4g

- Carbohydrates: 12g

- Fat: 14g

- Fiber: 3g

- Sugar: 6g

- Portion Size: 1 muffin

Banana Chocolate Chip Cookies

Ingredients:

- 2 ripe bananas, mashed

- 1/4 cup almond butter

- 1/4 cup maple syrup

- 1 teaspoon vanilla extract

- 1 1/2 cups rolled oats

- 1/4 cup dark chocolate chips

Instructions:

1. Preheat the oven to 350°F (175°C). Line a baking sheet with parchment paper.

2. In a mixing bowl, combine mashed bananas, almond butter, maple syrup, and vanilla extract.

3. Stir in rolled oats and chocolate chips until well combined.

4. Drop spoonfuls of the cookie dough onto the prepared baking sheet, spacing them apart.

5. Flatten each cookie slightly with the back of a spoon.

6. Bake for 12-15 minutes, or until the cookies are golden brown around the edges.

7. Allow the cookies to cool on the baking sheet for 5 minutes before transferring to a wire rack to cool completely.

Nutrition Information (per serving):

- Calories: 90
- Protein: 2g
- Carbohydrates: 13g
- Fat: 4g
- Fiber: 2g
- Sugar: 6g
- Portion Size: 1 cookie

Raspberry Coconut Truffles

Ingredients:

- 1 cup fresh raspberries

- 1/2 cup shredded coconut (unsweetened), plus extra for rolling
- 1/4 cup almond flour
- 2 tablespoons maple syrup
- 1/4 teaspoon vanilla extract

Instructions:

1. In a food processor, blend raspberries until smooth.
2. Transfer the raspberry puree to a mixing bowl and stir in shredded coconut, almond flour, maple syrup, and vanilla extract until well combined.
3. Roll the mixture into small balls using your hands.
4. Roll each ball in shredded coconut to coat.
5. Place the truffles on a plate or baking sheet lined with parchment paper.
6. Refrigerate for at least 30 minutes before serving.

Nutrition Information (per serving):

- Calories: 70
- Protein: 1g
- Carbohydrates: 7g
- Fat: 5g

- Fiber: 2g
- Sugar: 4g
- Portion Size: 1 truffle

Almond Butter Banana Bites

Ingredients:

- 2 ripe bananas, sliced
- 2 tablespoons almond butter
- 2 tablespoons chopped almonds

Instructions:

1. Spread almond butter on half of the banana slices.
2. Top with the remaining banana slices to make sandwiches.
3. Dip each banana bite into chopped almonds to coat the edges.
4. Place the banana bites on a plate or baking sheet lined with parchment paper.
5. Freeze for at least 1 hour before serving.

Nutrition Information (per serving):

- Calories: 90

- Protein: 2g

- Carbohydrates: 11g

- Fat: 5g

- Fiber: 2g

- Sugar: 6g

- Portion Size: 2 banana bites

Carrot Cake Energy Balls

Ingredients:

- 1 cup rolled oats

- 1/2 cup shredded carrots

- 1/4 cup almond butter

- 2 tablespoons maple syrup

- 1 teaspoon cinnamon

- 1/4 cup chopped walnuts

- 1/4 cup shredded coconut (unsweetened)

Instructions:

1. In a food processor, combine rolled oats, shredded carrots, almond butter, maple syrup, and cinnamon.

2. Pulse until the mixture comes together.

3. Transfer the mixture to a mixing bowl and stir in chopped walnuts and shredded coconut.

4. Roll the mixture into small balls using your hands.

5. Place the energy balls on a plate or baking sheet lined with parchment paper.

6. Refrigerate for at least 30 minutes before serving.

Nutrition Information (per serving):

- Calories: 80
- Protein: 2g
- Carbohydrates: 10g
- Fat: 4g
- Fiber: 2g
- Sugar: 4g
- Portion Size: 1 energy ball

Blueberry Almond Crisp

Ingredients:

- 2 cups fresh or frozen blueberries
- 1 tablespoon maple syrup
- 1 tablespoon lemon juice
- 1/2 cup almond flour

- 1/4 cup rolled oats

- 2 tablespoons coconut oil, melted

- 2 tablespoons chopped almonds

- 1 tablespoon coconut sugar (optional)

- Pinch of salt

Instructions:

1. Preheat the oven to 350°F (175°C). Grease a baking dish with coconut oil.

2. In a mixing bowl, toss blueberries with maple syrup and lemon juice. Transfer to the prepared baking dish.

3. In another bowl, combine almond flour, rolled oats, melted coconut oil, chopped almonds, coconut sugar (if using), and a pinch of salt. Mix until crumbly.

4. Sprinkle the almond-oat mixture evenly over the blueberries.

5. Bake for 25-30 minutes, or until the topping is golden brown and the blueberries are bubbling.

6. Allow the crisp to cool slightly before serving.

Nutrition Information (per serving):

- Calories: 120
- Protein: 2g
- Carbohydrates: 14g
- Fat: 7g
- Fiber: 3g
- Sugar: 8g
- Portion Size: 1/2 cup

Chocolate Covered Strawberries

Ingredients:

- 1 cup strawberries
- 1/4 cup dark chocolate chips
- 1 teaspoon coconut oil

Instructions:

1. Wash and dry strawberries, leaving the stems intact.
2. In a microwave-safe bowl, combine dark chocolate chips and coconut oil.
3. Microwave in 30-second intervals, stirring in between, until the chocolate is melted and smooth.

4. Dip each strawberry into the melted chocolate, coating about halfway up.

5. Place the dipped strawberries on a baking sheet lined with parchment paper.

6. Refrigerate for 10-15 minutes, or until the chocolate hardens.

7. Serve chilled.

Nutrition Information (per serving):

- Calories: 60
- Protein: 1g
- Carbohydrates: 8g
- Fat: 4g
- Fiber: 2g
- Sugar: 5g
- Portion Size: 2 strawberries

Mango Coconut Sorbet

Ingredients:

- 2 ripe mangoes, peeled and diced
- 1/2 cup coconut milk (canned, full-fat)
- 2 tablespoons maple syrup (optional)

- 1 tablespoon lime juice

- Pinch of salt

Instructions:

1. Place diced mangoes in a blender or food processor.

2. Add coconut milk, maple syrup (if using), lime juice, and a pinch of salt.

3. Blend until smooth and creamy.

4. Transfer the mixture to a shallow dish or ice cream maker.

5. If using a shallow dish, freeze for about 4 hours, stirring every hour until set.

6. If using an ice cream maker, follow the manufacturer's instructions.

7. Once frozen, scoop the sorbet into bowls and serve immediately.

Nutrition Information (per serving):

- Calories: 120

- Protein: 1g

- Carbohydrates: 22g

- Fat: 4g

- Fiber: 2g
- Sugar: 19g
- Portion Size: 1/2 cup

Chapter 7: Smoothies

In this chapter, we present refreshing and nutrient-rich smoothie recipes that are not only bursting with flavor but also designed to support your well-being. From vibrant green detox blends to indulgent chocolate-infused creations, there's a smoothie for every taste preference.

Green Detox Smoothie

Ingredients:

- 1 cup spinach leaves
- 1/2 cucumber, peeled and chopped
- 1/2 green apple, cored and chopped
- 1/2 lemon, juiced
- 1/2 inch fresh ginger, peeled
- 1 cup coconut water
- Ice cubes (optional)

Instructions:

1. Place all the ingredients in a blender.
2. Blend until smooth and creamy.

3. Add ice cubes if desired and blend again until well combined.

4. Pour into a glass and enjoy!

Nutrition Information:

- Calories: 120
- Protein: 3g
- Carbohydrates: 25g
- Fat: 1g
- Fiber: 6g
- Sugar: 15g
- Portion Size: 1 serving

Berry Blast Smoothie

Ingredients:

- 1 cup mixed berries (strawberries, blueberries, raspberries)
- 1/2 banana
- 1/2 cup almond milk
- 1/4 cup Greek yogurt (or dairy-free alternative)
- 1 tablespoon honey or maple syrup (optional)
- Ice cubes

Instructions:

1. Combine all the ingredients in a blender.

2. Blend until smooth and creamy.

3. Taste and adjust sweetness if necessary by adding honey or maple syrup.

4. Pour into a glass, garnish with fresh berries if desired, and serve.

Nutrition Information:

- Calories: 150
- Protein: 5g
- Carbohydrates: 30g
- Fat: 2g
- Fiber: 6g
- Sugar: 20g
- Portion Size: 1 serving

Mango Tango Smoothie

Ingredients:

- 1 ripe mango, peeled and diced
- 1/2 cup pineapple chunks
- 1/2 cup orange juice

- 1/2 cup coconut water

- 1/4 cup plain Greek yogurt (or dairy-free alternative)

- Ice cubes (optional)

Instructions:

1. Place all ingredients in a blender.

2. Blend until smooth and creamy.

3. Add ice cubes if desired and blend again until well combined.

4. Pour into a glass, garnish with a slice of mango, and enjoy!

Nutrition Information:

- Calories: 180

- Protein: 4g

- Carbohydrates: 40g

- Fat: 1g

- Fiber: 5g

- Sugar: 30g

- Portion Size: 1 serving

Peanut Butter Banana Smoothie

Ingredients:

- 1 ripe banana
- 2 tablespoons peanut butter
- 1 cup almond milk
- 1 tablespoon honey or maple syrup (optional)
- 1/2 teaspoon vanilla extract
- Ice cubes (optional)

Instructions:

1. In a blender, combine the banana, peanut butter, almond milk, honey or maple syrup, and vanilla extract.
2. Blend until smooth and creamy.
3. Add ice cubes if desired and blend again until well combined.
4. Pour into a glass, garnish with a drizzle of peanut butter, and serve.

Nutrition Information:

- Calories: 250
- Protein: 7g

- Carbohydrates: 30g

- Fat: 12g

- Fiber: 4g

- Sugar: 18g

- Portion Size: 1 serving

Tropical Paradise Smoothie

Ingredients:

- 1/2 cup pineapple chunks

- 1/2 cup mango chunks

- 1/2 banana

- 1/2 cup coconut milk

- 1/4 cup orange juice

- Ice cubes (optional)

Instructions:

1. Combine all ingredients in a blender.

2. Blend until smooth and creamy.

3. Add ice cubes if desired and blend again until well combined.

4. Pour into a glass, garnish with a pineapple slice, and enjoy!

Nutrition Information:

- Calories: 200
- Protein: 2g
- Carbohydrates: 35g
- Fat: 7g
- Fiber: 4g
- Sugar: 25g
- Portion Size: 1 serving

Kale Pineapple Smoothie

Ingredients:

- 1 cup chopped kale leaves, stems removed
- 1/2 cup pineapple chunks
- 1/2 banana
- 1/2 cup coconut water
- 1/4 cup plain Greek yogurt (or dairy-free alternative)
- Ice cubes (optional)

Instructions:

1. Place all ingredients in a blender.
2. Blend until smooth and creamy.

3. Add ice cubes if desired and blend again until well combined.

4. Pour into a glass, garnish with a kale leaf, and serve.

Nutrition Information:

- Calories: 140
- Protein: 6g
- Carbohydrates: 25g
- Fat: 2g
- Fiber: 5g
- Sugar: 15g
- Portion Size: 1 serving

Blueberry Almond Smoothie

Ingredients:

- 1/2 cup blueberries (fresh or frozen)
- 1/4 cup almonds
- 1/2 banana
- 1 cup almond milk
- 1 tablespoon honey or maple syrup (optional)
- Ice cubes (optional)

Instructions:

1. Combine all ingredients in a blender.

2. Blend until smooth and creamy.

3. Add ice cubes if desired and blend again until well combined.

4. Pour into a glass, sprinkle with crushed almonds, and serve.

Nutrition Information:

- Calories: 220
- Protein: 6g
- Carbohydrates: 25g
- Fat: 12g
- Fiber: 5g
- Sugar: 15g
- Portion Size: 1 serving

Chocolate Banana Protein Smoothie

Ingredients:

- 1 ripe banana
- 1 tablespoon cocoa powder
- 1 scoop plant-based protein powder

- 1 cup almond milk
- 1 tablespoon honey or maple syrup (optional)
- Ice cubes (optional)

Instructions:

1. In a blender, combine the banana, cocoa powder, protein powder, almond milk, and honey or maple syrup.
2. Blend until smooth and creamy.
3. Add ice cubes if desired and blend again until well combined.
4. Pour into a glass, sprinkle with a pinch of cocoa powder, and enjoy!

Nutrition Information:

- Calories: 250
- Protein: 20g
- Carbohydrates: 30g
- Fat: 5g
- Fiber: 6g
- Sugar: 15g
- Portion Size: 1 serving

Spinach Mango Smoothie

Ingredients:

- 1 cup spinach leaves
- 1/2 cup chopped mango
- 1/2 banana
- 1/2 cup coconut water
- 1/4 cup plain Greek yogurt (or dairy-free alternative)
- Ice cubes (optional)

Instructions:

1. Place all ingredients in a blender.
2. Blend until smooth and creamy.
3. Add ice cubes if desired and blend again until well combined.
4. Pour into a glass, garnish with a slice of mango, and serve.

Nutrition Information:

- Calories: 160
- Protein: 6g
- Carbohydrates: 30g
- Fat: 2g

*   Fiber: 5g

*   Sugar: 20g

*   Portion Size: 1 serving

Orange Creamsicle Smoothie

Ingredients:

*   1 orange, peeled and segmented

*   1/2 banana

*   1/2 cup Greek yogurt (or dairy-free alternative)

*   1/2 cup almond milk

*   1 tablespoon honey or maple syrup (optional)

*   Ice cubes (optional)

Instructions:

1. Combine all ingredients in a blender.

2. Blend until smooth and creamy.

3. Add ice cubes if desired and blend again until well combined.

4. Pour into a glass, garnish with an orange slice, and serve.

Nutrition Information:

- Calories: 180
- Protein: 8g
- Carbohydrates: 35g
- Fat: 3g
- Fiber: 4g
- Sugar: 25g
- Portion Size: 1 serving

Papaya Coconut Smoothie

Ingredients:

- 1 cup diced papaya
- 1/2 cup coconut milk
- 1/2 cup pineapple chunks
- 1/2 banana
- 1/4 cup plain Greek yogurt (or dairy-free alternative)
- Ice cubes (optional)

Instructions:

1. In a blender, combine the papaya, coconut milk, pineapple chunks, banana, and Greek yogurt.
2. Blend until smooth and creamy.

3. Add ice cubes if desired and blend again until well combined.

4. Pour into a glass, garnish with shredded coconut, and enjoy!

Nutrition Information:

- Calories: 220
- Protein: 5g
- Carbohydrates: 35g
- Fat: 8g
- Fiber: 6g
- Sugar: 20g
- Portion Size: 1 serving

Avocado Spinach Smoothie

Ingredients:

- 1/2 ripe avocado
- 1 cup spinach leaves
- 1/2 cup pineapple chunks
- 1/2 cup almond milk
- 1 tablespoon honey or maple syrup (optional)
- Ice cubes (optional)

Instructions:

1. Place all ingredients in a blender.

2. Blend until smooth and creamy.

3. Add ice cubes if desired and blend again until well combined.

4. Pour into a glass, garnish with a slice of avocado, and serve.

Nutrition Information:

- Calories: 200

- Protein: 5g

- Carbohydrates: 30g

- Fat: 10g

- Fiber: 6g

- Sugar: 20g

- Portion Size: 1 serving

Peach Ginger Smoothie

Ingredients:

- 1 cup sliced peaches (fresh or frozen)

- 1/2 inch fresh ginger, peeled and grated

- 1/2 cup almond milk

- 1/4 cup plain Greek yogurt (or dairy-free alternative)

- 1 tablespoon honey or maple syrup (optional)

- Ice cubes (optional)

Instructions:

1. Combine all ingredients in a blender.

2. Blend until smooth and creamy.

3. Add ice cubes if desired and blend again until well combined.

4. Pour into a glass, garnish with a slice of peach, and serve.

Nutrition Information:

- Calories: 180

- Protein: 6g

- Carbohydrates: 30g

- Fat: 3g

- Fiber: 5g

- Sugar: 20g

- Portion Size: 1 serving

Cherry Vanilla Smoothie

Ingredients:

- 1 cup pitted cherries (fresh or frozen)
- 1/2 cup vanilla-flavored almond milk
- 1/2 cup Greek yogurt (or dairy-free alternative)
- 1 tablespoon honey or maple syrup (optional)
- Ice cubes (optional)

Instructions:

1. In a blender, combine the cherries, almond milk, Greek yogurt, and honey or maple syrup.
2. Blend until smooth and creamy.
3. Add ice cubes if desired and blend again until well combined.
4. Pour into a glass, garnish with a cherry on top, and enjoy!

Nutrition Information:

- Calories: 200
- Protein: 7g
- Carbohydrates: 35g
- Fat: 3g

- Fiber: 5g
- Sugar: 25g
- Portion Size: 1 serving

Watermelon Mint Smoothie

Ingredients:

- 1 cup diced watermelon
- 1/4 cup fresh mint leaves
- 1/2 cup coconut water
- 1/2 cup Greek yogurt (or dairy-free alternative)
- 1 tablespoon honey or maple syrup (optional)
- Ice cubes (optional)

Instructions:

1. Place all ingredients in a blender.
2. Blend until smooth and creamy.
3. Add ice cubes if desired and blend again until well combined.
4. Pour into a glass, garnish with a sprig of mint, and serve.

Nutrition Information:

- Calories: 150
- Protein: 6g
- Carbohydrates: 30g
- Fat: 2g
- Fiber: 4g
- Sugar: 20g
- Portion Size: 1 serving

CONCLUSION

Congratulations on completing your journey through "Plant-Based Recipes for Diabetics to Manage Blood Sugar." Throughout this book, we've embarked on a flavorful and nutritious exploration of plant-based cooking tailored specifically to support individuals managing diabetes. From hearty breakfasts to satisfying dinners, from energizing smoothies to delightful desserts, each recipe has been carefully crafted to not only tantalize your taste buds but also to help stabilize your blood sugar levels.

By adopting a plant-based diet rich in whole grains, legumes, fruits, vegetables, nuts, and seeds, you've taken a proactive step towards better health and well-being. These recipes are not just about managing diabetes; they're about embracing a lifestyle that nurtures your body, mind, and spirit. With each meal, snack, and sip, you're nourishing yourself with the vibrant colors and flavors of nature's bounty.

As you continue on your plant-based diabetic journey beyond these pages, remember the principles that have guided you here. Listen to your body, experiment with new ingredients and flavors, and most importantly, enjoy the process. Whether you're cooking for yourself, your family, or friends, share the love and joy that comes from preparing wholesome, delicious meals together.

Your commitment to a plant-based lifestyle is not only benefiting your own health but also contributing to a healthier planet. By reducing your reliance on animal products and supporting sustainable food choices, you're making a positive impact on the environment and future generations.

As you savor the last bite of your favorite recipe from this book, know that this is just the beginning of your culinary adventure. Embrace the abundance of plant-based ingredients around you, and let your creativity flourish in the kitchen. Thank you for joining us on this flavorful journey, and may your path to wellness be filled with delicious moments and vibrant health.

Bon appétit and happy cooking!